Colon Cancer:

Breaking the Taboo and Taking Control

By

Michael J. Mills

Table of contents

Introduction

If you or someone you love has been affected by colon cancer, you know just how scary and overwhelming the diagnosis can be. But you're not alone. In fact, colon cancer is the third most common cancer in both men and women, and it's estimated that over 100,000 new cases will be diagnosed in the United States this year alone.

Despite its prevalence, colon cancer is still a topic that many people are uncomfortable discussing openly. But the truth is, the more we talk about it, the more we can do to prevent and treat it. That's why this book aims to break the taboo surrounding colon cancer and provide you with the knowledge and resources you need to take control of your health.

In these pages, you'll find a wealth of information about colon cancer, including its causes, symptoms, and risk factors. We'll also explore the various screening and diagnostic tests that are available, as well as the latest treatments and therapies. Along the way, we'll hear from survivors and experts in the field who will share their insights and experiences with you.

But this book is more than just a guide to colon cancer. It's also a roadmap for taking control of your health and well-being. We'll discuss lifestyle changes you can make to reduce your risk of developing colon cancer, as well as ways to cope with the emotional and psychological challenges that come with a diagnosis.

At its core, "Colon Cancer: Breaking the Taboo and Taking Control" is a message of hope. With the right knowledge, tools, and support, you can take an active role in managing your colon health and fighting this disease. So let's get started and break the taboo together.

Chapter 1: Colon Cancer an Overview and Its Stages

Colon cancer, also known as colorectal cancer, is a type of cancer that affects the large intestine or rectum. It is the third most common cancer in both men and women, and it's estimated that over 100,000 new cases will be diagnosed in the United States this year alone.

The exact causes of colon cancer are not fully understood, but it is believed to develop from polyps or abnormal growths that form on the lining of the colon or rectum. Over time, these polyps can become cancerous and spread to other parts of the body.

Colon cancer often does not cause symptoms in its early stages, which is why regular screening is so important. Common symptoms that may develop as the disease progresses include changes in bowel habits, blood in the stool, abdominal pain or discomfort, and unexplained weight loss.

Treatment for colon cancer will depend on the stage of the disease and other individual factors such as age, overall health, and medical history. Options may include surgery to remove the cancerous tissue, radiation therapy, chemotherapy, or a combination of these approaches.

There are also many lifestyle factors that can impact a person's risk of developing colon cancer, such as diet, exercise, and smoking habits. Maintaining a healthy lifestyle and following recommended screening guidelines can help to reduce your risk of developing colon cancer and improve your overall health.

If you have been diagnosed with colon cancer or are concerned about your risk, it's important to work closely with your healthcare team to develop a personalized treatment plan that meets your individual needs. With early detection and proper treatment, many people with colon cancer are able to successfully overcome the disease and live healthy, fulfilling lives.

Stages of Colon Cancer

Colon cancer is classified into different stages, depending on how far the cancer has spread. Understanding the stages of colon cancer is important in determining the appropriate treatment plan for each individual. In this chapter, we'll explore the different stages of colon cancer and what they mean for your diagnosis and treatment.

Stage 0 Colon Cancer:

At this stage, the cancer cells are still localized within the innermost lining of the colon and have not spread to other tissues or organs. Stage 0 colon cancer is often discovered during routine colonoscopies, and it is highly treatable with a high survival rate. In most cases, the recommended treatment for stage 0 colon cancer is surgery to remove the affected tissue or endoscopic removal. If the cancer is not completely removed during the first procedure, additional surgery may be necessary.

Stage I Colon Cancer:

At this stage, the cancer has grown through the innermost layer of the colon and into the next layer of tissue but has not yet spread to nearby lymph nodes or other organs. Treatment for stage I colon cancer typically involves surgery to remove the affected section of the colon. In some cases, a portion of the surrounding healthy tissue may also be removed. This is called a partial colectomy. After surgery, some individuals may require additional chemotherapy or radiation therapy to reduce the risk of the cancer returning.

Stage II Colon Cancer:

At this stage, the cancer has spread beyond the inner layers of the colon and into the muscle layer or the outermost layer of tissue, but has not yet spread to nearby lymph nodes or other organs. Treatment for stage II colon cancer usually involves surgery to remove the affected tissue, followed by chemotherapy or radiation therapy, or a combination of both. In some cases, individuals with stage II colon cancer may not require additional treatment after surgery.

Stage III Colon Cancer:

At this stage, the cancer has spread to nearby lymph nodes but has not yet spread to other parts of the body. Treatment for stage III colon cancer may include surgery to remove the affected tissue and nearby lymph nodes, followed by chemotherapy to kill any remaining cancer cells. The goal of treatment for stage III colon cancer is to reduce the risk of the cancer coming back and to improve the individual's chances of long-term survival.

Stage IV Colon Cancer:

At this stage, the cancer has spread to other parts of the body, such as the liver or lungs. Treatment for stage IV colon cancer may involve surgery to remove the affected tissue and radiation therapy to help control the growth of the cancer. Chemotherapy and targeted therapies may also be used to slow the growth of the cancer and improve quality of life. While treatment for stage IV colon cancer may not cure the cancer, it can help to prolong the individual's life and improve their overall quality of life.

Understanding the different stages of colon cancer is important in determining the appropriate treatment plan for each individual. If you have been diagnosed with colon cancer, it's important to work closely with your healthcare team to develop a personalized treatment plan that meets your individual needs. Early detection and treatment of colon cancer can greatly improve your chances of long-term survival and a better quality of life.

Chapter 2: Types of Cancer

Colorectal cancer is a term used to describe both colon and rectal cancers, but these two types of cancer are actually quite different in terms of diagnosis, treatment, and prognosis. Let's take a closer look at each type of cancer:

Colon Cancer:

Colon cancer, also known as colorectal cancer, is a type of cancer that starts in the colon or large intestine. The colon is the part of the digestive system that absorbs water and nutrients from food and stores waste until it is eliminated from the body. The most common type of colon cancer is adenocarcinoma, which develops from the cells that line the inside of the colon. Other less common types of colon cancer include carcinoid tumors, gastrointestinal stromal tumors (GISTs), and lymphomas.

Rectal Cancer:

Rectal cancer is a type of cancer that starts in the rectum, which is the last 6 inches of the large intestine that connects to the anus. Like colon cancer, rectal cancer most often develops from the cells that line the inside of the rectum, but it can also develop from other types of cells, such as those that produce hormones. The most common type of rectal cancer is adenocarcinoma.

Other Types of Colorectal Cancer:

In addition to colon and rectal cancers, there are other types of colorectal cancer that are less common but still important to know about. These include:

1.   Anal cancer: a type of cancer that starts in the anus, which is the opening at the end of the rectum through which waste is eliminated from the body.

2.   Carcinoid tumors: a rare type of cancer that can develop in the digestive tract, including the colon and rectum. Carcinoid tumors usually grow slowly and may not cause symptoms for many years.

3.   Gastrointestinal stromal tumors (GISTs): a type of tumor that can develop in the muscle or connective tissue of the digestive tract. GISTs are rare, but they can be aggressive and difficult to treat.

4.   Lymphomas: a type of cancer that develops in the lymphatic system, which is a network of tissues and organs that help the body fight infection. Lymphomas that start in the colon or rectum are rare.

It's also important to note that within each type of colorectal cancer, there are different subtypes that can affect the prognosis and treatment options. For example, adenocarcinomas can be categorized as either well-differentiated or poorly differentiated, with the latter being more aggressive and harder to treat. Additionally, rectal cancer can be divided into two categories based on its location: upper rectal cancer, which is closer to the colon, and lower rectal cancer, which is closer to the anus. The location of the cancer can affect the type of surgery that is needed and the likelihood of preserving bowel function.

Another important aspect to consider is the stage of the cancer. Colorectal cancer is staged from 0 to IV, with stage 0 being the earliest and stage IV being the most advanced. The stage of the cancer is determined by the size of the tumor, whether it has spread to nearby lymph nodes, and whether it has metastasized to other parts of the body. Knowing the stage of the cancer is critical in determining the appropriate treatment plan and predicting the patient's prognosis.

Treatment options for colorectal cancer vary depending on the type and stage of the cancer. Surgery is often the primary treatment for localized cancer, with the goal of removing the tumor and surrounding tissue. Chemotherapy and radiation therapy may also be used in combination with surgery to increase the chances of cure or control of the cancer. For advanced or metastatic cancer, chemotherapy and targeted therapies may be used to slow the progression of the disease and improve quality of life.

While colon and rectal cancers are the most common types of colorectal cancer, there are other types of cancer that can also affect the digestive system. Understanding the different types of colorectal cancer is important in determining the appropriate treatment plan for each individual. If you have been diagnosed with colorectal cancer, it's important to work closely with your healthcare team to develop a personalized treatment plan that meets your individual needs. Early detection and treatment of colorectal cancer can greatly improve your chances of long-term survival and a better quality of life.

Causes of Colon Cancer

Colorectal cancer is a complex disease that develops from a combination of genetic and environmental factors. Although the exact causes of colon cancer are not yet fully understood, research has identified several risk factors that can increase the likelihood of developing this type of cancer.

1.   Age: One of the most significant risk factors for colon cancer is age. The risk of developing colon cancer increases after the age of 50, with the majority of cases occurring in people over the age of 60.

2.   Genetics: Inherited genetic mutations can increase the risk of developing colon cancer. In particular, mutations in genes such as APC, MLH1, and MSH2 are associated with an increased risk of developing hereditary nonpolyposis colorectal cancer (HNPCC), also known as Lynch syndrome. Other genetic syndromes, such as familial adenomatous polyposis (FAP), can also increase the risk of developing colon cancer.

3.   Personal or family history of colon cancer: Individuals who have previously had colon cancer are at a higher risk of developing a new colon cancer than those who have never had the disease. Additionally, individuals who have a family history of colon

cancer, particularly in first-degree relatives such as parents or siblings, are also at an increased risk of developing the disease.

4.   Diet and lifestyle: A diet high in red and processed meats, saturated fats, and low in fiber can increase the risk of developing colon cancer. Additionally, a sedentary lifestyle, obesity, and smoking have all been associated with an increased risk of developing colon cancer.

5.   Inflammatory bowel disease: Individuals with a history of inflammatory bowel disease (IBD), such as ulcerative colitis or Crohn's disease, are at an increased risk of developing colon cancer. The risk

increases with the duration and severity of the disease.

6.   Radiation exposure: Exposure to high levels of radiation, such as during radiation therapy for other types of cancer, can increase the risk of developing colon cancer.

7.   Environmental factors: Exposure to certain environmental factors, such as air pollution or industrial chemicals, may increase the risk of developing colon cancer. However, the extent to which environmental factors play a role in the development of colon cancer is still unclear.

Researchers continue to investigate the underlying causes of colon cancer, and new risk factors are being identified. For example, recent studies have shown that disruptions in the gut microbiome, the collection of bacteria and other microorganisms that live in the digestive tract, may play a role in the development of colon cancer. Changes in the gut microbiome have been linked to inflammation and alterations in the immune system, which can contribute to the development of cancer.

Other potential risk factors that are currently being studied include the use of nonsteroidal anti-inflammatory drugs (NSAIDs), such as aspirin, and the use of antibiotics. Studies have suggested that long-term use of NSAIDs may reduce the risk of developing colon cancer, possibly by reducing inflammation in the colon. However, the use of NSAIDs can also have side effects, so individuals should discuss the risks and benefits with their healthcare provider before using these medications for colon cancer prevention.

Similarly, while antibiotics are often used to treat infections, there is some evidence to suggest that they may also alter the gut microbiome and increase the risk of developing colon cancer. More research is needed to fully understand the relationship between antibiotics and colon cancer, but individuals should be cautious about using antibiotics unnecessarily.

While the exact causes of colon cancer are not fully understood, research has identified several risk factors that can increase the likelihood of developing this disease. By understanding these risk factors, individuals can take steps to reduce their risk of developing colon cancer. This may include making dietary and lifestyle changes, such as maintaining a healthy weight, eating a diet high in fruits and vegetables, and engaging in regular physical activity. Additionally, individuals with a personal or family history of colon cancer may benefit from increased screening and monitoring by their healthcare provider.

Chapter 3: Symptoms of Colon Cancer

Colon cancer often develops without any noticeable symptoms in its early stages, which is why routine screening is so important. However, as the cancer grows and progresses, it can cause a range of symptoms that may indicate the presence of the disease. Here are some common symptoms of colon cancer:

1.   Changes in bowel habits: One of the most common symptoms of colon cancer is a change in bowel habits, such as diarrhea, constipation, or a change in the consistency of stools.

2. Blood in the stool: Colon cancer can cause bleeding in the rectum or colon, which may be visible as blood in the stool. Blood may appear as bright red, dark red, or black, depending on where in the digestive tract the bleeding is occurring.

3. Abdominal pain or discomfort: Colon cancer can cause pain or discomfort in the abdomen, which may be mild or severe. This pain may be persistent or come and go.

4. Fatigue: Colon cancer can cause fatigue or weakness, which may be caused by anemia or the body's immune response to the cancer.

5.   Unexplained weight loss: Colon cancer can cause unexplained weight loss, which may occur as a result of a loss of appetite or changes in the way the body absorbs nutrients.

6.   Nausea and vomiting: Colon cancer can cause nausea and vomiting, particularly if the cancer is causing a blockage in the digestive tract.

7.   Iron deficiency anemia: Colon cancer can cause chronic blood loss in the digestive tract, which can lead to iron deficiency anemia. This may cause symptoms such as fatigue, weakness, and shortness of breath.

8.   Obstruction: As the tumor grows, it can cause a blockage in the colon,

leading to symptoms such as abdominal pain, bloating, and nausea.

9. Bowel perforation: In rare cases, colon cancer can cause a hole or perforation in the wall of the colon, which can lead to infection and other serious complications.

10. Spread to other organs: If colon cancer spreads to other organs, it can cause a range of symptoms depending on the location of the metastases. For example, if the cancer spreads to the liver, it may cause jaundice, abdominal pain, and weight loss.

It is important to note that not everyone with colon cancer will experience symptoms, and some individuals may have advanced-stage cancer before any symptoms develop. This is why regular screening is so important, especially for individuals with a personal or family history of colon cancer.

It is also important to note that these symptoms can be caused by a variety of conditions other than colon cancer, such as hemorrhoids or inflammatory bowel disease. However, if you are experiencing any of these symptoms, it is important to talk to your healthcare provider to determine the underlying cause and receive appropriate treatment.

Remember that early detection and treatment can improve outcomes for individuals with colon cancer. If you are at average risk for colon cancer, you should begin screening at age 50 or earlier if you have a family history of the disease or other risk factors. Screening tests such as colonoscopies and stool tests can detect colon cancer in its early stages, when treatment is most effective.

In summary, while colon cancer may not cause noticeable symptoms in its early stages, it can cause a range of symptoms as it progresses. It is important to be aware of these symptoms and to speak with your healthcare provider if you are experiencing any of them. Regular screening is also important for early detection and treatment of colon cancer, especially for individuals with a personal or family history of the disease.

Chapter 4: Risk Factors

While anyone can develop colon cancer, there are certain factors that can increase an individual's risk of developing the disease. Some of these risk factors are modifiable, meaning that they can be changed or managed, while others are non-modifiable. Here are some of the most common risk factors for colon cancer:

1.   Age: The risk of colon cancer increases with age, with the majority of cases occurring in individuals over age 50.

2.   Personal history of colon cancer or polyps: Individuals   who   have

previously had colon cancer or certain types of polyps are at an increased risk of developing the disease.

3.   Family history of colon cancer: Individuals with a family history of colon cancer are at an increased risk of developing the disease themselves, especially if the family member was diagnosed at a young age.

4.   Inflammatory bowel disease: Individuals with a history of inflammatory bowel disease, such as Crohn's disease or ulcerative colitis, are at an increased risk of developing colon cancer.

5.   Sedentary lifestyle: Lack of physical activity and a sedentary

lifestyle have been linked to an increased risk of colon cancer.

6. Obesity: Being overweight or obese has been linked to an increased risk of colon cancer.

7. Smoking: Smoking has been linked to an increased risk of colon cancer, as well as many other types of cancer.

8. Alcohol consumption: Heavy alcohol consumption has been linked to an increased risk of colon cancer.

3333333ë9. Diet: A diet high in red and processed meats, and low in fruits, vegetables, and fiber, has been linked to an increased risk of colon cancer.

It is important to note that having one or more of these risk factors does not necessarily mean that an individual will develop colon cancer. However, individuals with one or more risk factors should talk to their healthcare provider about appropriate screening and lifestyle modifications to reduce their risk of developing the disease.

While some risk factors for colon cancer cannot be changed, such as age and family history, there are steps that individuals can take to reduce their risk of developing the disease. These include:

1. Maintaining a healthy weight: Being overweight or obese has been linked to an increased risk of colon

cancer. By maintaining a healthy weight through regular exercise and a healthy diet, individuals can reduce their risk.

2.   Eating a healthy diet: A diet high in fiber, fruits, and vegetables, and low in red and processed meats, has been linked to a reduced risk of colon cancer. It is also important to limit alcohol consumption and avoid smoking.

3.   Regular screening: Regular screening for colon cancer is important, especially for individuals with a personal or family history of the disease. Screening tests such as colonoscopies and stool tests can detect colon cancer in its early stages when treatment is most effective.

4.	Managing inflammatory bowel disease: Individuals with inflammatory bowel disease, such as Crohn's disease or ulcerative colitis, should work with their healthcare provider to manage their condition and reduce their risk of developing colon cancer.

5.	Discussing risk with healthcare provider: Individuals with one or more risk factors for colon cancer should talk to their healthcare provider about appropriate screening and risk reduction strategies.

By taking these steps, individuals can reduce their risk of developing colon cancer and improve their overall health. It is important to remember that early detection and treatment can improve outcomes for individuals with colon cancer, so regular screening is essential for early detection. By working with their healthcare provider and making healthy lifestyle choices, individuals can take control of their colon cancer risk and live healthier lives.

Chapter 5: Diagnosis of Colon Cancer

Colon cancer can be diagnosed through a variety of tests and procedures. Early detection is important for successful treatment, as colon cancer is most treatable in its early stages. Here are some of the most common diagnostic tests and procedures for colon cancer:

1.   Colonoscopy: Colonoscopy is a procedure that uses a thin, flexible tube with a camera on the end to examine the inside of the colon. During a colonoscopy, polyps can be removed for biopsy and cancer can be diagnosed.

2.   Biopsy: A biopsy is a procedure that involves removing a small piece of tissue for examination under a microscope. If a polyp is found during a colonoscopy, a biopsy can be done to determine if it is cancerous.

3.   Stool tests: Stool tests are used to detect blood or other abnormalities in the stool that may indicate the presence of colon cancer.

4.   Imaging tests: Imaging tests, such as CT scans, MRIs, and X-rays, can be used to detect the presence of colon cancer and determine its size and location.

5.   Blood tests: Blood tests can be used to detect certain markers that may indicate the presence of colon cancer.

If colon cancer is diagnosed, additional tests may be needed to determine the stage of the cancer and whether it has spread to other parts of the body. Staging is important for determining the best course of treatment and predicting outcomes. Staging may involve additional imaging tests, such as PET scans, and biopsies of nearby lymph nodes.

It is important for individuals to talk to their healthcare provider about appropriate screening tests for colon cancer based on their age, risk factors, and medical history. Early detection is key to successful treatment, so it is important to be aware of the symptoms of colon cancer and to seek medical attention if they occur. With prompt diagnosis and appropriate treatment, individuals with colon cancer can improve their outcomes and live healthier lives.

In addition to these diagnostic tests and procedures, it is important to note that individuals with a personal or family history of colon cancer may be at increased risk for the disease. In these cases, genetic counseling and testing may be recommended to identify any inherited genetic mutations that may increase the risk of colon cancer. Genetic testing can also help guide treatment decisions and screening recommendations for individuals with a higher risk of developing colon cancer.

It is important for individuals to work closely with their healthcare provider to determine the most appropriate diagnostic tests and screening recommendations based on their individual risk factors and medical history. By staying informed and proactive about colon cancer screening and diagnosis, individuals can improve their chances of early detection and successful treatment.

It is also important to note that while a colon cancer diagnosis can be scary and overwhelming, there are a variety of treatment options available, including surgery, chemotherapy, radiation therapy, and targeted therapy. These treatments can help shrink tumors, prevent the spread of cancer, and improve outcomes for individuals with colon cancer. Support groups and counseling services can also be helpful resources for individuals and their families coping with a colon cancer diagnosis. With the right care and support, individuals with colon cancer can improve their quality of life and achieve positive outcomes.

Chapter 6: Treatment of Colon Cancer

Treatment for colon cancer depends on several factors, including the stage of the cancer, the location and size of the tumor, and the overall health of the individual. Here are some of the most common treatments for colon cancer:

1.   Surgery: Surgery is often the first line of treatment for colon cancer. During surgery, the tumor and surrounding tissue are removed. In some cases, a portion of the colon may need to be removed as well. In more advanced cases, surgery may also involve removing nearby lymph nodes or other affected organs.

2. Chemotherapy: Chemotherapy uses drugs to kill cancer cells throughout the body. It is often used after surgery to kill any remaining cancer cells and reduce the risk of recurrence. Chemotherapy can also be used in combination with radiation therapy for more advanced cases of colon cancer.

3. Radiation therapy: Radiation therapy uses high-energy beams of radiation to kill cancer cells. It is often used in combination with chemotherapy for more advanced cases of colon cancer.

4. Targeted therapy: Targeted therapy is a type of treatment that uses drugs to target specific proteins or genes that

contribute to the growth of cancer cells. This treatment can be effective in treating advanced cases of colon cancer.

5. Immunotherapy: Immunotherapy is a newer type of treatment that helps the body's immune system fight cancer. It works by blocking proteins that prevent the immune system from attacking cancer cells.

6. Palliative care: Palliative care focuses on improving the quality of life for individuals with advanced or metastatic colon cancer. It may involve pain management, symptom relief, and emotional support.

It is important for individuals with colon cancer to work closely with their healthcare provider to determine the most appropriate treatment options based on their individual needs and medical history. Treatment may also involve a multidisciplinary team of healthcare professionals, including surgeons, oncologists, and radiation therapists.

While the prospect of treatment for colon cancer can be daunting, it is important to remember that there are many effective treatment options available. With the right care and support, individuals with colon cancer can improve their outcomes and achieve a better quality of life. It is also important to engage in regular follow-up care and monitoring to detect any potential recurrence of the cancer and address any ongoing symptoms or side effects of treatment.

It is important for individuals undergoing colon cancer treatment to take an active role in their care by staying informed, following their treatment plan, and communicating openly with their healthcare providers about any concerns or questions they may have. It is also important to maintain a healthy lifestyle during and after treatment, including eating a balanced diet, engaging in regular physical activity, and avoiding smoking and excessive alcohol consumption.

In addition to medical treatment, individuals with colon cancer may benefit from complementary therapies such as acupuncture, massage therapy, and meditation, which can help manage symptoms and promote relaxation and well-being.

It is important to note that while treatments for colon cancer can be effective, they can also have side effects. These may include fatigue, nausea, hair loss, and changes in bowel habits. It is important for individuals to discuss any potential side effects with their healthcare provider and to report any new or worsening symptoms.

Finally, it is important to remember that a colon cancer diagnosis can be difficult for individuals and their families, both emotionally and financially. Many individuals with colon cancer may experience anxiety, depression, and other psychological symptoms. Financial concerns may also arise due to the cost of medical treatment and time away from work. It is important to seek out support from loved ones, support groups, and healthcare providers to manage these challenges and achieve the best possible outcomes.

Outlook of Colon Cancer

The outlook for colon cancer depends on several factors, including the stage of the cancer at diagnosis, the location and size of the tumor, and the individual's overall health. In general, early detection and treatment can significantly improve the prognosis for individuals with colon cancer.

According to the American Cancer Society, the overall 5-year survival rate for colon cancer is approximately 90% for individuals whose cancer is diagnosed at an early stage. However, the 5-year survival rate decreases as the cancer progresses to more advanced stages. For example, the 5-year survival rate for individuals with stage III colon cancer is approximately 72%, while the rate for individuals with stage IV colon cancer is approximately 14%.

It is important to note that survival rates are based on statistics and do not necessarily reflect an individual's individual outcome. Each person's experience with colon cancer is unique, and the prognosis can vary depending on many individual factors.

Regular screening for colon cancer is essential for early detection and treatment. It is recommended that individuals begin screening for colon cancer at age 45, or earlier if they have certain risk factors such as a family history of colon cancer. Screening options include colonoscopy, fecal occult blood tests, and stool DNA tests.

In addition to regular screening, it is important for individuals to maintain a healthy lifestyle and manage any underlying medical conditions, as these can also affect the outlook for colon cancer. This includes eating a balanced diet, engaging in regular physical activity, avoiding smoking and excessive alcohol consumption, and managing any chronic health conditions such as diabetes or high blood pressure.

Finally, it is important for individuals with colon cancer to work closely with their healthcare providers to develop an appropriate treatment plan and to engage in regular follow-up care and monitoring. With the right care and support, individuals with colon cancer can improve their outcomes and achieve a better quality of life.

There are many lifestyle changes and supportive care strategies that can improve the outlook for individuals with colon cancer. These may include:

1.   Nutrition: Eating a healthy, balanced diet can help support the immune system and improve overall health. A diet rich in fruits, vegetables, whole grains, and lean proteins can also help manage symptoms such as fatigue, nausea, and constipation.

2.   Exercise: Regular physical activity can help improve energy levels, reduce stress, and manage symptoms such as fatigue and depression. Exercise may also help reduce the risk of colon cancer recurrence and improve overall quality of life.

3.   Support groups: Joining a support group can help individuals with colon cancer connect with others who are

going through similar experiences. This can provide emotional support, practical advice, and a sense of community.

4.   Palliative care: Palliative care is a specialized form of medical care that focuses on managing symptoms and improving quality of life for individuals with serious illnesses such as cancer. Palliative care may include pain management, counseling, and other supportive services.

5.   Clinical trials: Clinical trials are research studies that test new treatments or therapies for cancer. Participation in a clinical trial may provide access to new, cutting-edge treatments that are not yet widely available.

It is important to work closely with healthcare providers to develop an individualized treatment plan and to discuss any concerns or questions that may arise. With the right care and support, individuals with colon cancer can achieve the best possible outcomes and improve their overall quality of life.

Chapter 7: Prevention of Colon Cancer

While there is no guaranteed way to prevent colon cancer, there are several steps individuals can take to reduce their risk. These include:

1. Regular screening: Regular screening for colon cancer is one of the most effective ways to reduce the risk of developing the disease. Recommended screening options include colonoscopy, fecal occult blood tests, and stool DNA tests. The American Cancer Society recommends that individuals begin screening for colon cancer at age 45, or earlier if they

have certain risk factors such as a family history of colon cancer.

2. Healthy diet: A diet that is high in fiber, fruits, and vegetables, and low in red and processed meats, can help reduce the risk of colon cancer. It is also important to limit the intake of alcohol and avoid smoking.

3. Physical activity: Regular physical activity can help reduce the risk of colon cancer. The American Cancer Society recommends engaging in at least 150 minutes of moderate-intensity exercise or 75 minutes of vigorous-intensity exercise per week.

4. Maintain a healthy weight: Being overweight or obese can increase the

risk of colon cancer. Maintaining a healthy weight through regular exercise and a balanced diet can help reduce this risk.

5.   Manage chronic conditions: Certain chronic health conditions, such as inflammatory bowel disease, can increase the risk of colon cancer. Managing these conditions through regular medical care and treatment can help reduce the risk.

6.   Know your family history: Individuals with a family history of colon cancer may have an increased risk of developing the disease. It is important to talk to healthcare providers about family history and to follow recommended screening guidelines.

7.   Consider taking aspirin: For some individuals, taking a daily low-dose aspirin may help reduce the risk of colon cancer. However, it is important to talk to a healthcare provider before starting aspirin therapy, as it can increase the risk of bleeding and other side effects.

8.   Vitamin D: Some studies have suggested that low levels of vitamin D may be associated with an increased risk of colon cancer. It is important to talk to a healthcare provider about appropriate vitamin D supplementation.

9.   Reduce exposure to environmental toxins: Exposure   to   certain environmental toxins such as pesticides

and industrial chemicals may increase the risk of colon cancer. Taking steps to reduce exposure to these toxins, such as using natural cleaning products and avoiding smoking and secondhand smoke, may help reduce the risk.

10.   Hormone replacement therapy: Hormone replacement therapy (HRT) has been associated with an increased risk of colon cancer. It is important to talk to a healthcare provider about the potential risks and benefits of HRT, especially for individuals with a history of colon cancer or other risk factors.

11.   Genetic testing: In some cases, individuals may be at an increased risk of colon cancer due to inherited genetic mutations. Genetic testing can help

identify these individuals and guide appropriate screening and prevention measures.

By incorporating these additional steps into a comprehensive prevention plan, individuals can further reduce their risk of colon cancer and promote overall health and wellness. It is important to work closely with healthcare providers and to stay up-to-date on the latest research and recommendations regarding colon cancer prevention.

Next Step

If you have been diagnosed with colon cancer, it is important to work closely with healthcare providers to develop a personalized treatment plan. Treatment options for colon cancer may include surgery, chemotherapy, radiation therapy, targeted therapy, and immunotherapy. Healthcare providers will work with individuals to determine the best treatment plan based on factors such as the stage and location of the cancer, overall health and wellness, and personal preferences.

After treatment, it is important to engage in regular follow-up care to monitor for any signs of recurrence or new cancer. This may include regular imaging tests, blood work, and physical exams. Healthcare providers may also recommend lifestyle changes and preventive measures to reduce the risk of future cancer.

For individuals who have not been diagnosed with colon cancer, it is important to engage in regular screening and follow-up care as recommended by healthcare providers. By taking steps to reduce the risk of colon cancer, individuals can promote overall health and wellness and reduce the impact of this disease on their lives.

It is also important to stay informed and educated about colon cancer and to advocate for increased awareness and funding for research and prevention efforts. By working together as a community, we can make progress in the fight against colon cancer and improve outcomes for all individuals impacted by this disease.